THE STRANGE EGG

OTHER TITLES FROM THE EMMA PRESS

ART SQUARES

The Goldfish, by Ikhda Ayuning Maharsi Degoul, illustrated by Emma Dai'an Wright
Menagerie, by Cheryl Pearson, illustrated by Amy Evans
One day at the Taiwan Land Bank Dinosaur Museum, by Elīna Eihmane
Pilgrim, by Lisabelle Tay, illustrated by Reena Makwana
The Fox's Wedding, by Rebecca Hurst, illustrated by Reena Makwana

POETRY COLLECTIONS

Europe, Love Me Back, by Rakhshan Rizwan

POETRY PAMPHLETS

The Bell Tower, by Pamela Crowe
Ovarium, by Joanna Ingham
Milk Snake, by Toby Buckley

SHORT STORIES

Tiny Moons: A year of eating in Shanghai, by Nina Mingya Powles,
    illustrated by Emma Dai'an Wright
Postcard Stories 2, by Jan Carson, illustrated by Benjamin Phillips
Hailman, by Leanne Radojkovich
Night-time Stories, edited by Yen-Yen Lu

BOOKS FOR CHILDREN

My Sneezes Are Perfect, by Rakhshan Rizwan, illustrated by Benjamin Phillips
The Bee Is Not Afraid of Me: A Book of Insect Poems, edited by Fran Long
    and Isabel Galleymore, illustrated by Emma Dai'an Wright
Cloud Soup, by Kate Wakeling, illustrated by Elīna Brasliņa
Oskar and the Things, by Andrus Kivirähk, illustrated by Anne Pikkov,
    translated from Estonian by Adam Cullen

THE STRANGE EGG

A Symptoms Diary

KIRSTIE MILLAR

ILLUSTRATED BY HANNAH MUMBY

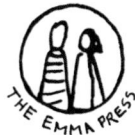

THE EMMA PRESS

'It is a strange realism, but it is a strange reality.'
– Ursula K. Le Guin, The Carrier Bag Theory of Fiction

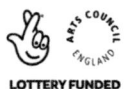

Supported using public funding by
ARTS COUNCIL ENGLAND
LOTTERY FUNDED

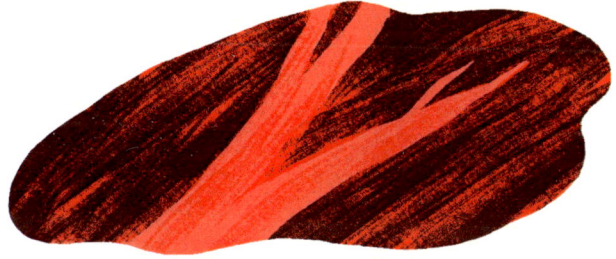

MENSTRUAL PHASE

(bleeding)

1.

Picture this: white fawn, spotless and new, running and suddenly punctured by a particularly sharp branch. Mother's salty tongue licking the wound clean.

Three drops of crimson blood steaming in the snow. Blood is terribly revealing. Blood for the hunters to see and also smell.

Picture this: the white fawn and its mother do not know the mistake they have made. Sadly, the hunter knows. Sadly, the sharp teeth always know.

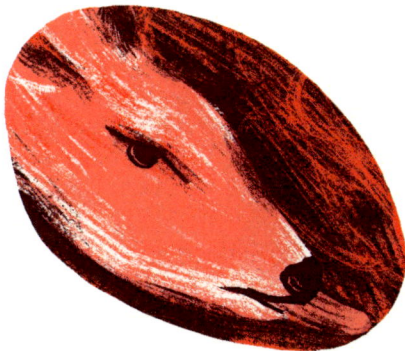

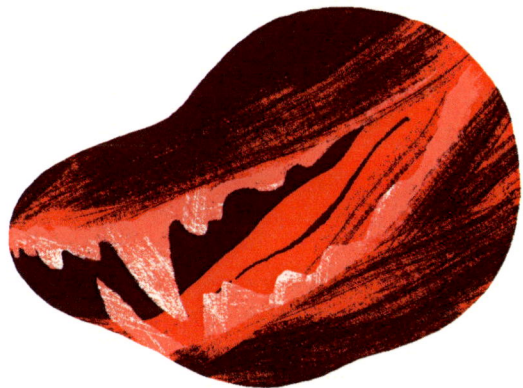

2.

The birth was painful. Like all births. This agony sprouted from my side and raged and raged.

    Me: on the bathroom floor.

    Me: crawling. All hands and knees and whimpers.

3.

Too much withering on the floor. Too much churning. Pain all guttural and hot.

Me: on your table. Legs parted and trembling in your hooks, naked from the waist down.

You: a blue-gloved hand inside of me. Tugging at the birth. Twisting the pain in your meaty fist. Flecks of blood against the white of your coat.

'For your own good,' you say.

'Okay,' I say. 'Okay.'

4.

(After the birth)

Doctor, I write this while bleeding in my little bed. I am sore. But I am feeling brighter today. I lean on my pillow and sip cups of tea with demerara sugar. Through my cracked window I smell cold winter sun. Decades of dust cling to my yellowed curtains.

I rent a small bedroom at the top of a large house on the edge of the city. The landlady is kind but odd. The house is full of fur coats; these quiet animals with button eyes hang limply on hooks. To reach my bedroom I must walk past the swaying animals, up and up a long and narrow stairwell on which a bright red rug stretches out like a tongue.

The landlady has many sons. They eat and fight and throw stones at cats and smoke cigarettes in the dishevelled garden beneath my window. I do not like her sons; they do not like me.

In the corner there is the birth. Fully formed and realised. A glowing egg.

5.

The egg cries all night. I cannot bear its noiseless sobs.
I rock the egg. I cover it with a blanket. I tell it a story.
I threaten to smash it with a spoon. Nothing
helps. Nothing stops the tortured cries.

The landlady hears my anxious
pacing feet and knocks on my door.
'What is the matter, dear?'

Knock. Knock.

'What are you hiding?'

Knock.

Knock.

I ignore her and then she leaves.

Doctor, I am very exhausted.
But I cannot sleep; the egg will
not allow it.

Perhaps you can give me something?

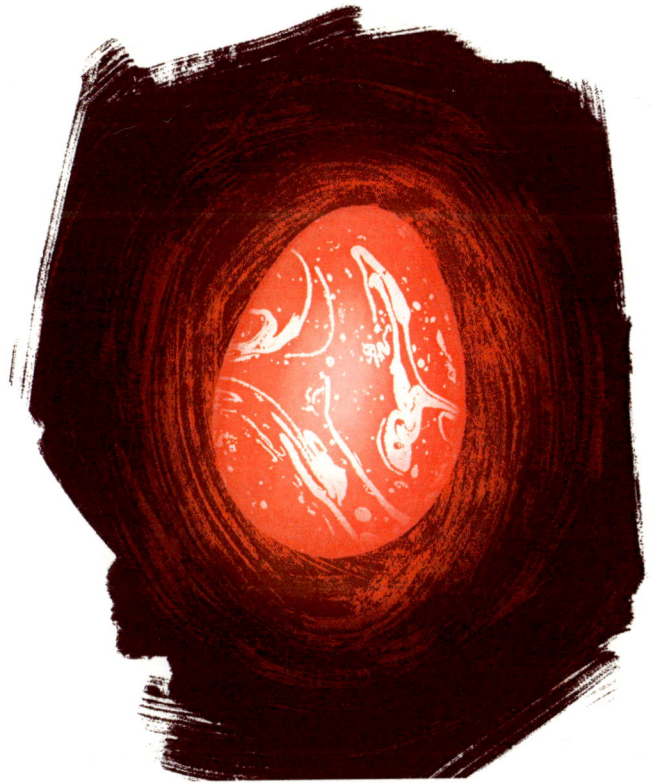

5

6.

I am overcome by a strange memory. Although I have tried to forget it, I cannot. So I leave the egg in the crate and walk and do not stop until I reach the woods.

The white fawn is here and I tell the fawn my memory:

> It is night and I am running. I am running wildly and purely; each tree whooshes past my ear and my body is compact and capable and strong. The trees and snow and sky smell delicious and promising and I am happy.

> Then suddenly a ripping, a hot damp heat splashing through my core. I feel pain with a sickening certainty.

> Agony, sharp and ancient, ruptures me.

> I stop my delightful running. Tending to my wound, I discover a gash has split me open. There is blood. Pulsing and chaotic and everywhere. I look down at the snow. See it is crimson, shimmering and horrible.

The fawn watches me with intelligent eyes and slowly chews grass.

> I ask the fawn: What is it like to be hunted, to be harmed?

7.

Doctor, I am still bleeding. Here are my new symptoms:

Blood runs from me furiously.

I pass clots. Black and as big as pennies.

A blue star ebbs viscously in my left eye.

Desperate to soothe myself, I climb into the bath and sigh as steaming water rises around me. The dull churning in my abdomen goes quiet. My bones throb, but more slowly.

I peer over the bath's edge and see the strange egg. Still lying in its little crate. Still so white and smooth and rotten.

I cannot stand the egg. I cannot stand its silence. I cannot stand its sickening cries. How it watches me.

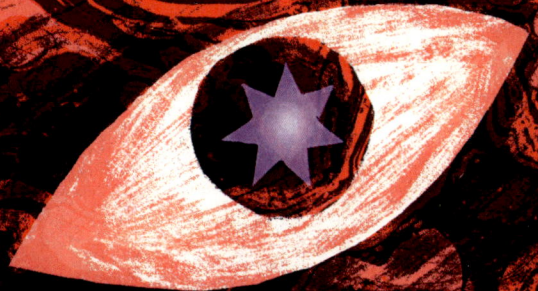

8.

(Night)

I leave my house and walk purposefully down the sleeping road.

> The egg: malicious and twisted and wrong.

> Me: clutching the egg in my arms, my legs slick. Droplets fall from my body and burn the snow.

From beneath the grate the sewer twinkles and moves rapidly, a quick pulse of the underworld.

> Me: on my knees, pulling back the grate, hands trembling around the shell, bone cold and ominous and then, suddenly, gone!

> The egg: appears like an opal swept away by the foaming current. Furious at this abandonment.

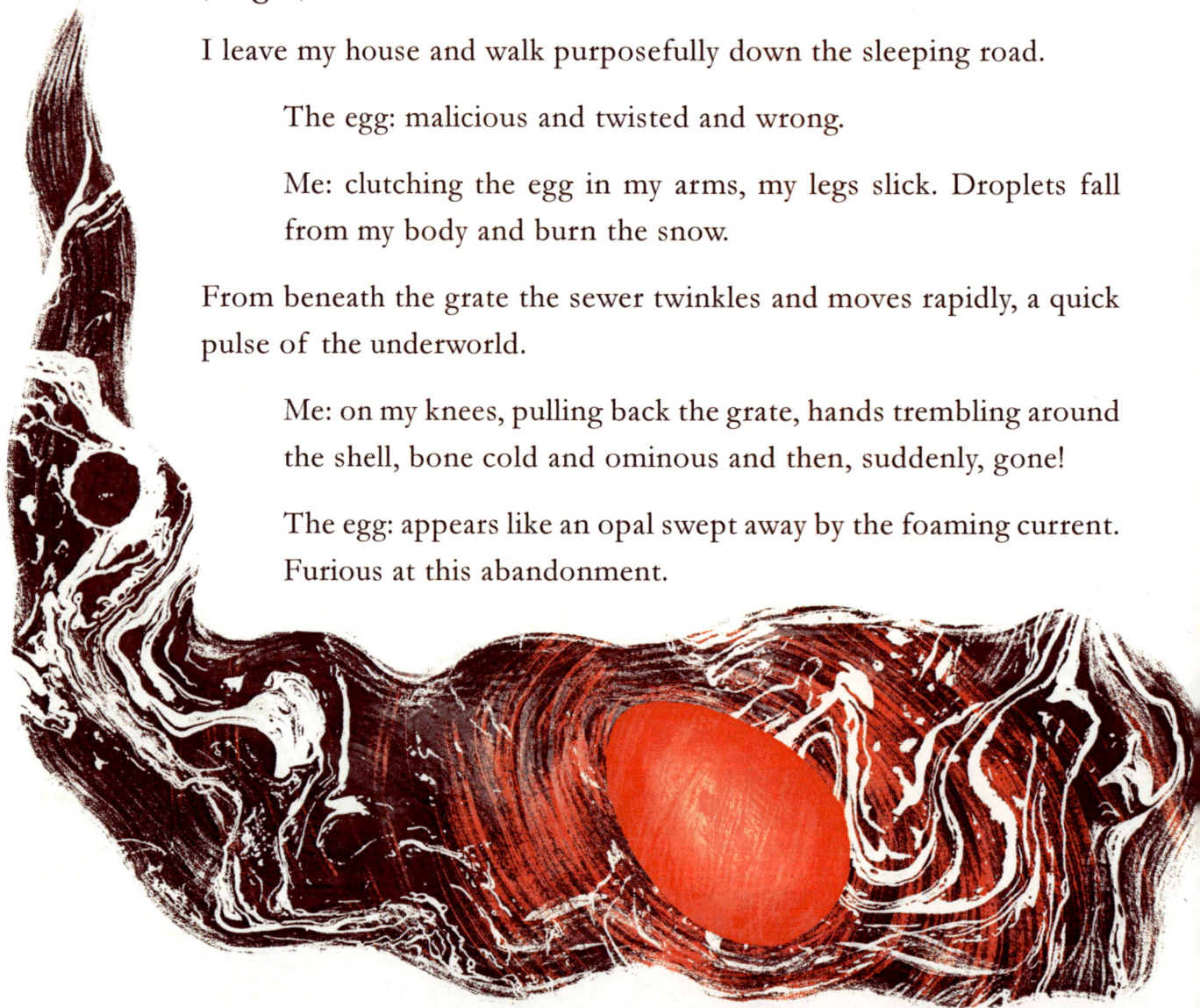

FOLLICULAR PHASE

9.

Doctor, my bleeding has stopped! I luxuriate in this freedom, eat bread dipped in milk, bone-white and steaming in the pot. My room is silent and delicious.

In town I visit the market and dresses flutter in the breeze. I admire their colours and picture myself wearing each one. I look at baskets of shining fruit and cheerful sticks of bread. I buy an apple and a cinnamon bun, and the market seller playfully winks his bright eye at me.

I see a bowl of white eggs and my shopping smashes on the ground and I scream and scream and scream.

10.

Today my egg is impatient.

At the café a woman brings back a cup of coffee and points angrily at the mug. 'The coffee is hot! The coffee is too hot!' the woman is yelling at me.

All day I serve piles of buttered toast and pastries with little cherries on top and ham sandwiches dripping with yellow mustard.

I say 'Thank you, please come again!' and count loose change and sweep floors while my egg screeches out in protest. I want to yell, *I hear you, egg!* I want to soothe it. I want to stomp on it, destroy it. I want to be free from it. But I cannot.

I do the washing-up. Pain burns viciously along my nerves. Tugs at my hips. Cloys sharply at my tender flesh.

Yes, I am concerned. But I try very hard to not think about the egg.

11.

I wake and the sky is a hollow blue. Today I am not hurting. The quiet in my body is gentle and expansive; it brings me to tears.

12.

(Work)

I am well I say to the floorboards with the snaggle nails as I run the brush over I am wellI say to the oven and the burnt bread and charred animal fat which I scrape like tiny corpses away from the cast iron I am well I say as the oven whines and moans in protest I am well I say to the windows which I wash with hot water and vinegar I am well I am well I am well!

With stinging hands, I gather dirty plates and cups. My stomach quivers with emptiness.

My body is light and malleable. The whole world flickers across my rolling eyes and I am gone.

I return to my body, surprised to discover myself limp and splayed across the café floor. Customers flutter over me, concerned and nervous. My boss is angry with me for fainting.

I am sent home early. My wages are docked.

13.

Let's see the white fawn.

[Picture this: The fresh point of the antlers hurt the baby skull. I know this shattering pain. But the white fawn bears it.]

The antlers appear – one for balance, one for perception.

It is winter for the fawn. There is so much frost underfoot and the ice can be deceptive. The fawn knows the frost, knows its quiet, devious language.

Me: by the frozen stream, which hums patiently.

The fawn: tender and conversational.

Me: hand outstretched and hopeful.

The fawn and I touch gently. Fingertip to nose. Then I ask the fawn about the wound – it seems the polite thing to do.

The wound is very painful. It bleeds and bleeds. Mother's tongue licks it clean. The blood stops. The blood comes back again.

OVULATION PHASE

(egg release)

14.

Doctor, I had a terrible dream.

In my dream I saw my own body, and I saw what you will do to it.

15.

(The Hospital)

A nurse greets me at the desk. Her cheeks are dusted pink and her mouth is brimming with large, luminous teeth.

I am handed a small plastic jar and directed to the bathroom. I carefully collect my urine in the jar and return it to the smiling nurse. My face burns. She instructs me to take a seat.

Waiting room sign: Be courteous. Be patient.

The egg: vivid and alive.

In the corner of the waiting room a woman rocks a baby and the baby cries.

16.

(Examination Room)

You call me into a dark room. You instruct me to undress from the waist down. The nurse yanks a curtain and I watch the leaning shadow of your back.

I step into a breezy paper gown and climb onto a narrow bed.

You emerge from behind the curtain, humming a little song as you squirt shimmering gel onto a pulsing wand. Without warning, you bluntly insert the wand inside of me. A small agony ripples out across my flesh; I try very hard not to scream.

> Doctor (cold eyes narrowing and darting across the screen): How very strange. It appears you have another egg.

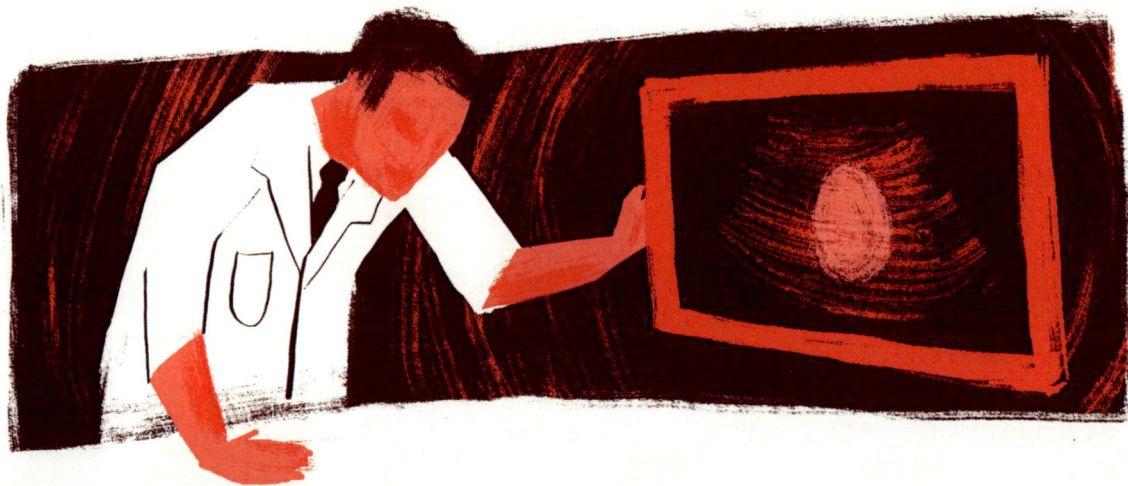

My heart is quick and sick in my chest! I try to run but cannot move.

The nurse is now over me; she grips my wrist tightly, her sharp pink nails pinching my skin, her bright teeth erupted into an impossible smile.

Doctor: Be still. Let's not be silly now. We aren't quite finished yet.

I obediently lie back on the bed. Tears thud furiously onto my blue paper gown and my legs shake wildly.

Doctor: There's a good girl. Now, would you like to see your egg?

Everything appears black and watery and eternal. But then your gloved finger traces something. I lean closer and I see it:

A strange new egg. Engorged and vicious. Humming with delight.

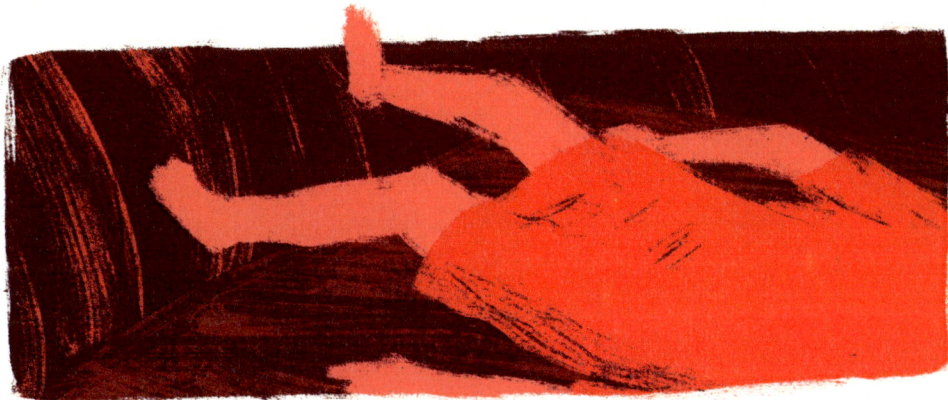

17.

Doctor, today there is a shifting.

A sudden blossoming inside me.

Rage? Yes, rage.

LUTEAL PHASE

(after egg release)

18.

(Town)

I wear long dresses to hide my disease, but soon my abdomen swells so large old women begin to smile at me meddlesomely.

Old woman (stretching out a wrinkled hand): Oh, how joyful!

I have been sent to buy cartons of milk for the café, and I wait in line at the shop. The cartons lie dumb and heavy in my tired arms.

Old woman: A boy or a girl?

Overcome with rage I wail. I say: *'No! No! I am not having a baby! I am diseased! I am swollen because of a terrible egg!'*

Shocked, the old woman stares back at me blankly. Then, understanding my words, she yanks her hand from the swell of my stomach and runs from the shop.

19.

(In the woods)

Despite best intentions, the mother's tongue cannot undo nature's brutality.

The fawn: injured and bleeding; little drips pant redly into snow.

Despite the frost I find meadowsweet. I drip honey onto the wound, sore and sadly festering.

The mother: paces watchfully, unhappy and desperate and mournful.

The fawn: does not cry out, does not protest, does not run in fear, but instead offers me great gentleness. Nudges my hand with a twitching nose, grazes my cold fingers with the antlers.

Together we eat apples. I pull dried chamomile from my bag, encouraging the fawn to bite the quiet yellow flowers. Lots of chewing.

The fawn and the mother abruptly sprint away.

20.

(At night)

I dream of a large black dog. Or is it white. Or is it without colour.

The dog: teeth sinking further into my secret flesh. Lips licking. Taunting laughter.

No, not me! Yes, me. Well, a part of me.

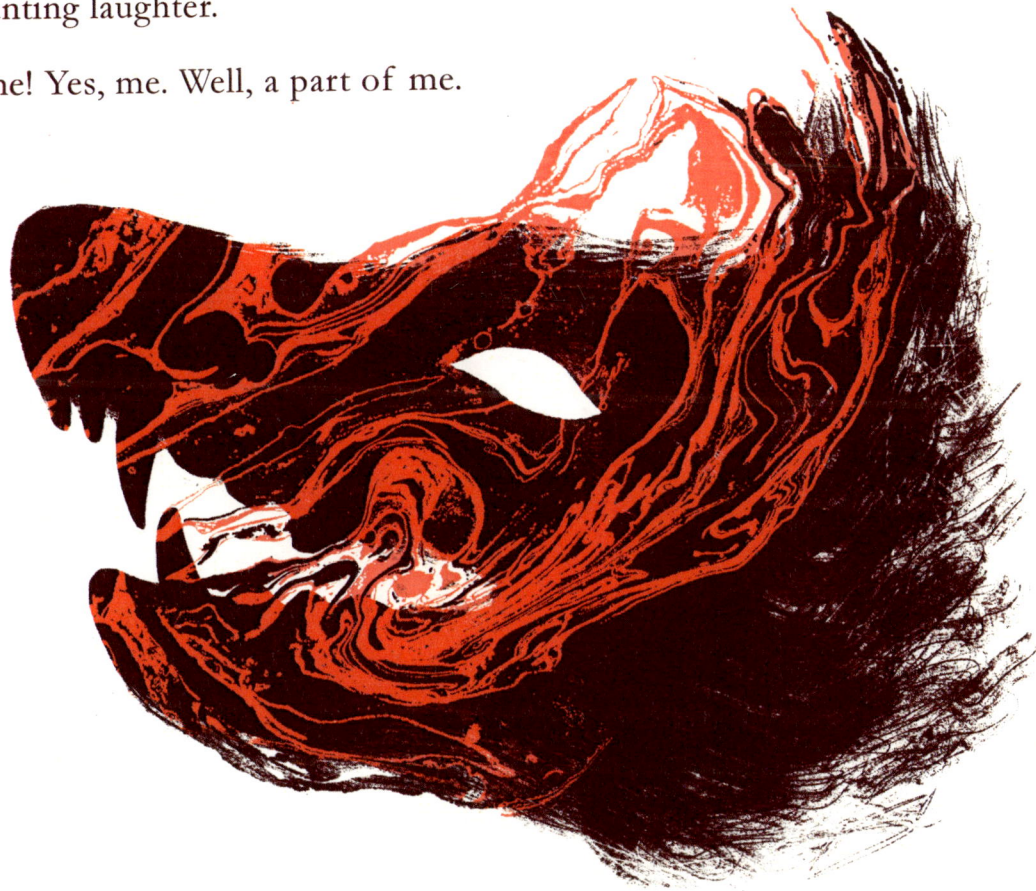

21.

(A follow-up appointment)

You prescribe me fresh air. You prescribe me a hobby. You prescribe more meat in my diet.

> Me: I am confined to my wretched bed. I am teeming with sickness and night sweat.

> I wake to find myself wounded. Abdomen scraped at, strips of skin dangling lifelessly from my red nails. Frantic, bloody crescents.

> Doctor: Do not dwell!

> Me: But how am I meant to live like this?

> Doctor: The pain is yours. Nothing can be done. You must bear it.

(Inside of me)

The new egg. A bigger, stronger disease.

22.

Today the egg has grown larger and more malevolent.

Overcome with bright and thundering pain, I flee my yellow room.

>Me: tumbling down the dark stairs.

>My disease: seeps across organs, amniotic and wet.

Pain is wild and clear like a vision. I tread around consciousness. I encounter little pockets of darkness. Realise that death is like a puddle.

My thoughts are white mice. My thoughts leap and fall. My thoughts skitter stupidly from light to pain to light again.

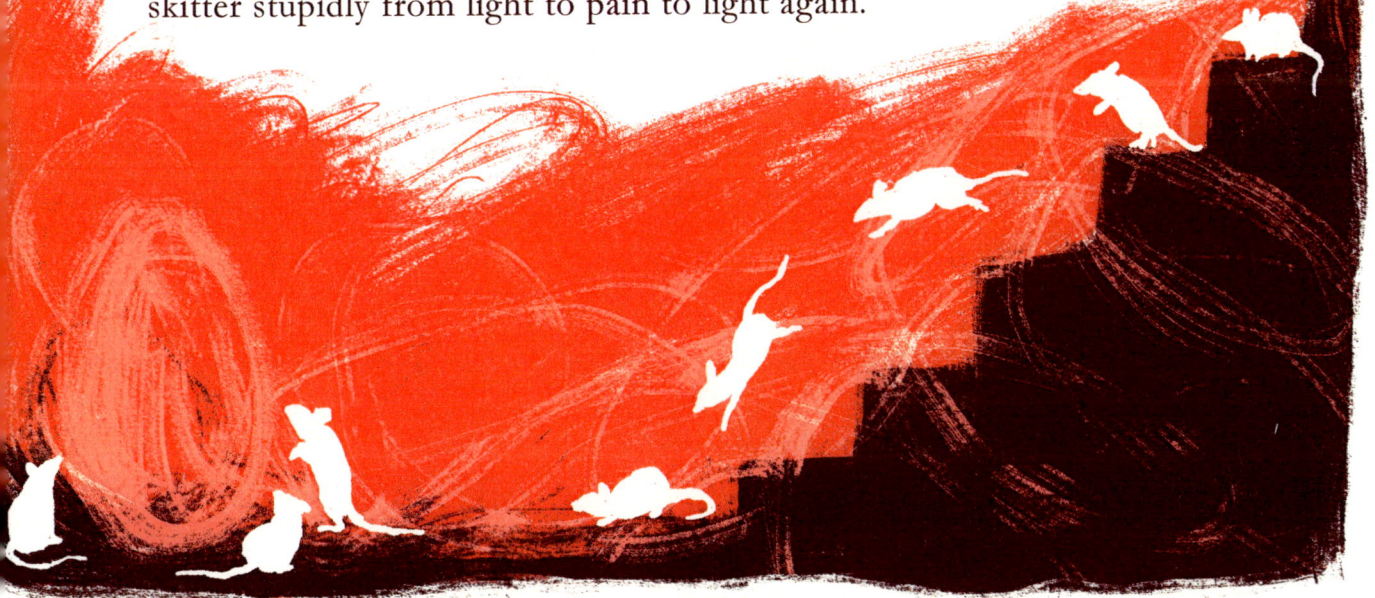

23.

(The bottom of the stairs)

The landlady's son eventually discovers me, crumpled and bleeding. He stands closer, leans over me. I grasp his hand, wrap my arms around his leg and beg him to free me from the egg.

He looks down at me with pity. But upon seeing my terrible blood, seeping and crimson and everywhere, he lurches away, mortified.

Doctor, you are called.

24.

(Operating theatre)

I find myself on your table. Awake and frantic and screaming.

Doctor: indifferent, eyes lupine and glinting

Me: teeth bared, clawing like an animal at your white coat

Doctor: plunges a needle into the pillow of my blue vein

Me: feel as if wading backwards through cold water

Doctor: undressing me, pinching limbs between fingertips, hooking my bare feet into metal stirrups

Me: languid and slack-jawed

Doctor: panting from behind your mask, dashes a scalpel across my abdomen, smiles as flesh melts away from blade

Me: my wounds moan

Doctor: wrist-deep inside the cavity of my abdomen, your hand up between my legs

Me: lifeless and indifferent

25.

I lunge back into bright and painful consciousness. Find myself wounded and bent in a hospital bed, a mask at my face, a drip embedded in my tender vein. My blood runs ominously. Forms a terrible river, ruins the starch-white sheets.

I yank back the blanket and lift up my gown to reveal myself. I am a shocking mess of bruises. Mottled and purple and clinging to crimson gashes. I am hastily stitched with a crust of black wire, tied into coarse little bows.

My abdomen butchered, rippled and seeping. I hurt deeply and eternally. My body weeps.

Suddenly, I hear crying. Mortified little wails. Sobs lurching in the soft flesh of the throat. My throat? Yes, yes. My throat.

Scorched from the tube and the howling.

26.

(After)

I do not want the scorching tea or stale toast which the nurse brings me. Her smile is still impossible, her dusted cheeks so pink and bright it makes me dizzy.

Me: I am so sore. How am I meant to live like this?

The nurse: The pain is yours; you must bear it.

Me: Was the surgery a success?

The nurse: What a silly question! No it was not! You know it never could be.

In the corner I see the strange egg. Pearlescent and diseased and watching. Waiting for me to rise and tend to it. Waiting to consume me.

27.

Nudged by some gentle force, I wake.

> The fawn: leans over my bed, tenderly licks blood from my face and my fingertips.

I rise. My abdomen half-slaughtered, my legs shaking and ungainly. The tiles are cold and solid beneath my feet. The hospital is all but abandoned. The fawn gallops wildly and I follow with slow determination.

We are fleeing. No one stops us.

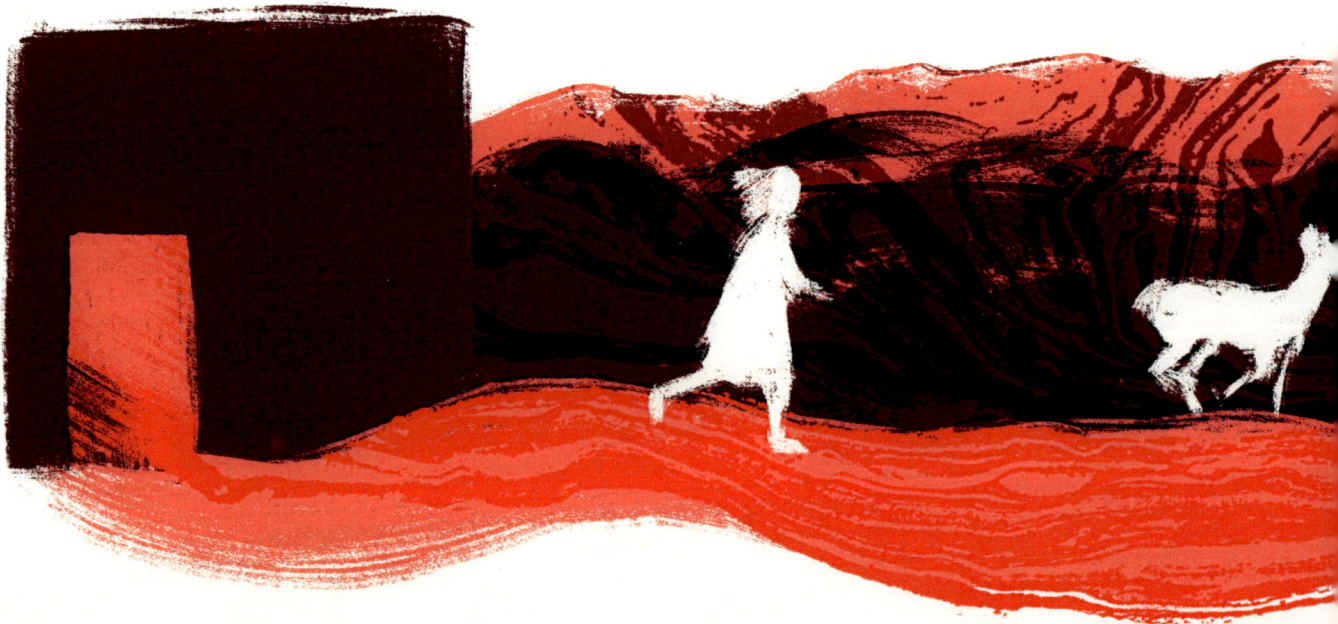

28.

Picture this: my blood as a trail. My blood as a rope. My blood as a ladder. My blood shimmering and bold, declaring my escape.

Outside it is clean and glorious. I limp behind the fawn as if newly born. We go further until my body rages in pain and my wounds pulse. We go further and further until we reach our joyous destination.

The woods twitch with life, with gentleness, with abundant possibility. The trees engulf us gladly. We are received with great kindness.

Doctor, I am still weak and hazy from your needle.

But my body, truthfully an animal, remembers.

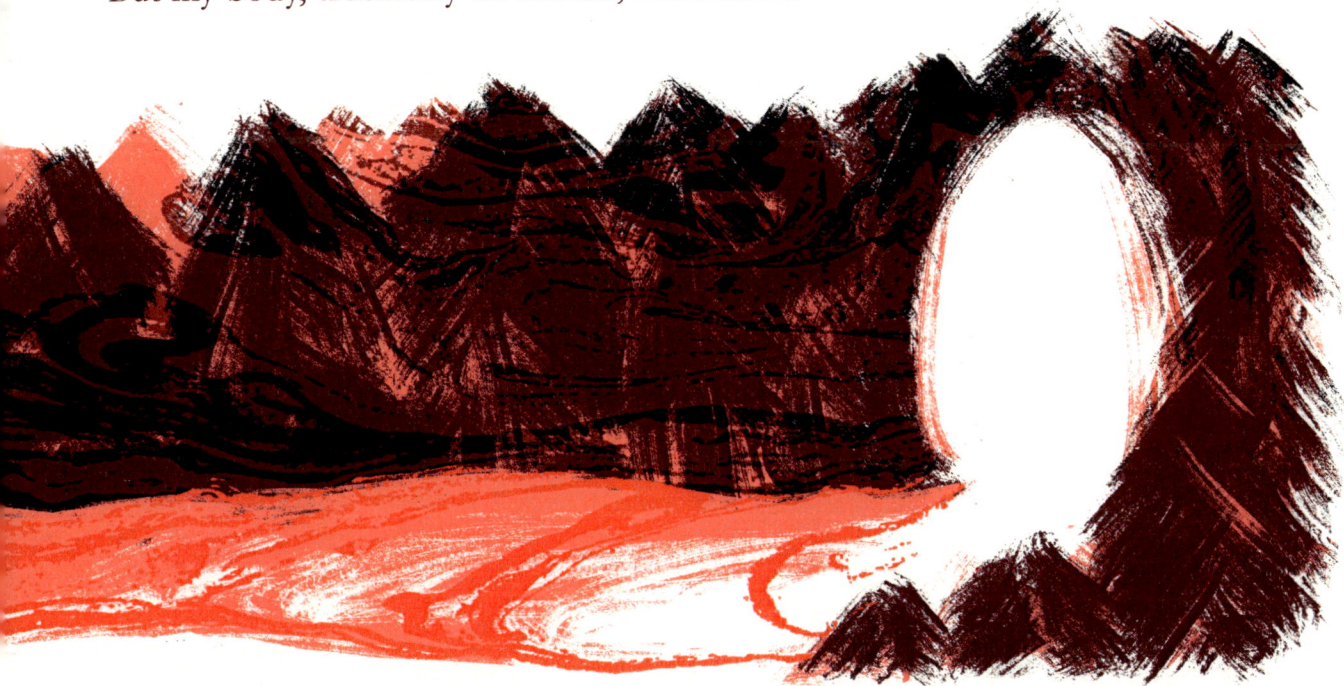

ACKNOWLEDGEMENTS

Thanks to my dear friends who live with chronic illness and pain.

Thank you to my teachers: Sandy Pool, for your insight and expertise as I developed *The Strange Egg* and Rebecca Tamàs, for your encouragement and guidance when I began writing poetry.

Thank you to Kate Birch, the Ink Sweat & Tears Scholarship made it possible for me to study and write this work on the MA in Creative Writing (Poetry) at UEA.

Thank you to Pema, Emma and the team at The Emma Press for choosing to publish *The Strange Egg*, and to Hannah Mumby, whose magical illustrations brought this story to life.

Thank you to my family, in particular my sister Danni and my mother Linda, for your love and friendship.

Finally, thank you to Theo, my husband and my best friend, for everything.

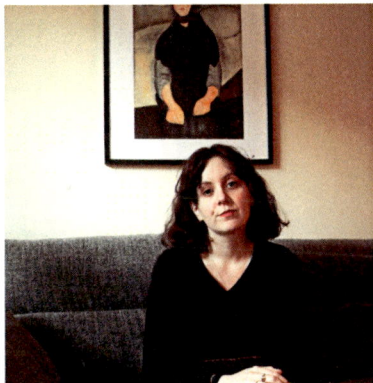

ABOUT THE AUTHOR

Kirstie Millar is a writer based in Manchester. In 2017 she founded *Ache*, an intersectional feminist press publishing writing and art on illness, health, bodies and pain. She completed her MA in Creative Writing at UEA and was a recipient of the Ink, Sweat and Tears Scholarship.

Her writing has been published by Prototype, 3 of Cups Press and has been commended by Penguin's WriteNow programme in 2020 and the UEA New Forms Awards in 2021.

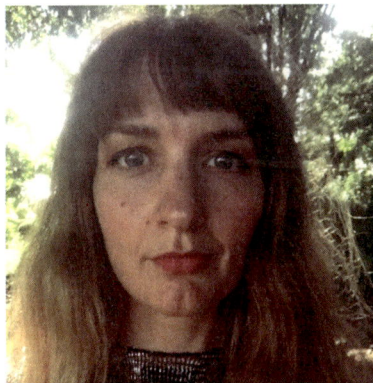

ABOUT THE ILLUSTRATOR

Hannah Mumby is an illustrator and artist based in south west England. Hannah's approach to illustration is rooted in paying close attention to the stories that we tell about ourselves, listening for subtle hidden meanings and associations. Her illustrations seek to open up new ways of reflecting on the narratives we are reading, and draw attention to mysterious or surreal threads that may be hidden beneath the surface. See more of Hannah's work at www.hannahmumby.co.uk

ABOUT THE EMMA PRESS

The Emma Press is an independent publishing house based in the Jewellery Quarter, Birmingham, UK. It was founded in 2012 by Emma Dai'an Wright, and specialises in poetry, short fiction and children's books.

The Emma Press has been shortlisted for the Michael Marks Award for Poetry Pamphlet Publishers in 2014, 2015, 2016, 2018, and 2020, winning in 2016.

In 2020 The Emma Press received funding from Arts Council England's Elevate programme, developed to enhance the diversity of the arts and cultural sector by strengthening the resilience of diverse-led organisations.

website: theemmapress.com
facebook: @theemmapress
twitter: @TheEmmaPress
instagram: @theemmapress